The
Drug-Free
Sleep
Solution

The 4-Week Program for Overcoming Insomnia
Using Cognitive Behavioral Therapy

David Durocher

Erikson Publishing

Copyright © 2021 by David Durocher.

Library of Congress Cataloging-in-Publication Data is Available.

ISBN-13: 9798742295648

Note: **The purpose of this book is to educate. It is not intended to serve as a replacement for professional medical advice. The author and publisher of the information in this book make no medical claims for its use. This material is intended to help you to get restful sleep on a regular basis using only cognitive-behavioral therapy. If you need medical attention, please consult your doctor. Neither the author nor the publisher is responsible for any injury caused directly or indirectly by the information contained in this book. The**

Contents

Introduction

Basic Facts about Sleep and Insomnia

Congratulations! You will soon be well on your way to getting the restful sleep that you deserve!

Getting enough quality sleep is very important for our mental, emotional, spiritual and physical health. It is linked to the quality of our relationships, our well-being, and our productivity. Insomnia is a common sleep disorder. In America today, 1 in 3 adults experience intermittent insomnia, while at least 1 in 10 experience chronic insomnia[1]. The American Sleep Disorders Association has stated that: "Of all the medical conditions today, few are as wide-ranging and as little understood as sleep disorders[2]." Insomnia is linked to motor accidents, decreased quality of life, diminished work productivity, and increased long-term risk for medical and psychiatric diseases[3]. It now rivals obesity and smoking as our greatest health hazard[4].

The NTSB (National Transportation Safety Board) estimates that fatigue contributes to as much as 25 percent of all transportation accidents--whether car, bus, truck, train, or plane. That statistic sounds shocking, but experts have known the truth for years. In 2011, the Centers for Disease Control and Prevention (CDC) declared insufficient sleep a public health epidemic--a warning on a par with those released about tobacco decades ago. "Sleep-deprived is the new normal, like smoking was in the 1950's," says Russell Sanna, PhD, former executive director of the Division of Sleep Medicine at Harvard Medical School[4]. The health risks of chronic insomnia may include: hypertension, diabetes, heart attack, depression, obesity (due to cortisol) and stroke[5].

According to a Harvard study conducted by Charles Czeisler in 2004[6], "One in twenty medics have confessed to making a mistake due to tiredness that it resulted in the death of a patient." Then there are the societal costs of insomnia in terms of lost productivity at work, and the personal cost of strained relationships and a lack of enjoyment of life[6]." Furthermore, a lack of adequate sleep may result in irritability, cognitive impairment, memory loss, and impaired moral judgement[5]. Depression and irritability, common symptoms of insomnia, are a leading cause of a phenomenon called "presenteeism", in which workers show up for their jobs but are incapable of doing productive work, costing the U.S. companies over $150 billion in lost productivity[7].

It's no coincidence that this insomnia phenomenon correlates with a decreased quality of life for Americans. Historically, America has been labeled as being "the greatest nation on earth." However, despite living in a democracy, America is not the greatest nation in terms of overall happiness.

According to the 2018 World Happiness Report, "Finland is the happiest country in the world[8]. The report ranks countries on six key variables that support well-being: income, freedom, trust, healthy life expectancy, social support and generosity. (The World Happiness Report was written by a group of independent experts acting in their personal capacities). 'The

top five countries all have almost equally high values for the six

factors found to support happiness, and four of these countries –

Denmark, Switzerland, Norway and now Finland – have been in

first place in the six World Happiness Report rankings since the

first report,' said report co-editor John Helliwell, a professor

emeritus of economics at the University of British Columbia[8]."

According to the World Happiness Report (U.N.), for the years

2016-2018, the United States was ranked #19 in the world[65].

According to Psychology Today ©, "Anecdotal information

suggests that life satisfaction can be distilled down to four

fundamental zones that define and provide meaning to our lives:

"**work**, **play**, **love**, and **prayer**[9]." For most people, these are the

pillars that support a stable, balanced and fulfilling life.

Evidently, a lot of people in the United States have not struck the

balance among these areas that many foreign people have. Or it

may just be that America has been stuck in a deep hole of

materialism for a very long time. We are wrong to think or

believe that we need things to be happy. The overall benefit of

new technology is now in question. It is no wonder that our

country has insomnia problems when you look at all of the

electronic gadgets and video game consoles that we buy and use

constantly. What remains is the sad fact that most people never

get the proper treatment for insomnia.

Insomnia is defined as either persistent difficulty in falling

asleep, or staying asleep or early-morning awakenings with

inability to return to sleep, or some combination of the three.

Insomnia is measured both subjectively and objectively. The

amount of quality sleep needed somewhat varies among

individuals[10]. Some people may need only 5 hours of quality of

sleep, while others may need as much as 10 hours. Most adults,

however, need 7 to 8 hours of quality sleep[10]. The bottom-line is

that if you require 8 hours of sleep and are only getting 6, then

you are not going to feel as well. In fact, you are far more likely

to feel moody and irritable. Furthermore, the longer you go without sleep, the more your brain will force sleep…the pressure just builds up.

There are two types of insomnia: primary and secondary. Secondary insomnia, today, is referred to as "comorbid insomnia." Current research is focused mainly on comorbid insomnia. This program, however, is indicated for both primary and comorbid insomnia.

Primary insomnia is sleeplessness without any medical, psychological, or environmental cause. The underlying causes of primary insomnia can be divided into the three following subgroups: **psychophysiological**, **idiopathic,** and **sleep state misperception**[11].

Psychophysiological insomnia is when a person with previous sleep adequacy, starts to experience sleeplessness because of a prolonged period of stress. The tension and anxiety from the stress causes awakening. Thereafter, sleep in such persons becomes associated with frustration and arousal, resulting in poor sleep hygiene. In most people, as the initial stress decreases, normal sleep habits are gradually restored because the bad sleep habits are not reinforced. However, in some people, the bad habits are reinforced, the person "learns" to worry about his or her sleep, and sleeplessness continues for years after the stress has subsided. Therefore, it is also called learned insomnia or behavioral insomnia.

Then there is **idiopathic insomnia**, which is a lifelong sleeplessness and is attributed to an abnormality in the neurologic control of the sleep-wake cycle involving areas of the brain responsible for wakefulness and sleep. It may begin in childhood. Those affected may have a dysfunction in the sleep state that predisposes the person towards arousal. Insomnia tends to persist over the entire life span and can be aggravated by stress or tension.

Finally, there is **sleep state misperception**, in which the person complains of insomnia without objective evidence or symptoms of any sleep disturbance; sleep duration and quality are completely normal. They typically do not display daytime sleepiness or other signs of poor-quality sleep. These people may be described as having "sleep hypochondriasis."

Hypochondria is an anxiety disorder which is similar to obsessive-compulsive disorder or OCD. These people are predisposed or "wired" to believe something that is, in fact, irrational. In sleep hypochondriasis, a person may believe that he or she didn't get enough sleep and then he or she has a negative automatic thought such as "not getting enough sleep is going to ruin my life"--he or she will worry about it based only on subjective reasoning. Subsequently, this disorder can lead to anxiety and depression.

The key to overcoming sleep hypochondriasis is to break up this vicious cycle of worrying. Through CBT-I, these people can learn to do this by challenging their negative assumptions and negative automatic thoughts. Basically, stress and worry are the triggers for initiating and maintaining psychophysiological insomnia, while stress alone triggers idiopathic insomnia. In sleep state misperception, cognitive therapy is needed to challenge and overcome faulty, automatic negative thing[11].

Comorbid Insomnia

Secondary insomnia also known as **comorbid insomnia** is far more prevalent than primary insomnia[12].

According to the American Sleep Association™ © 2015, the problems that can cause comorbid insomnia include:

- Certain illnesses, such as some heart and lung diseases.

- Pain disorders such as fibromyalgia.

- Medicines that delay or disrupt sleep as a side-effect.

- Caffeine, tobacco, alcohol, and other substances that affect sleep.

- Another sleep disorder such as restless legs syndrome or sleep apnea.

- A poor sleep environment.

- A change in sleep routine.

- Mental illness such as moderate to severe anxiety and/or depression, bipolar disorder, and schizophrenia.

People with psychiatric problems are far more likely to have insomnia than any other group in the general population.[12]. This group of people are far more likely to use or require medication.

A Personal Note

At the age of 19, during my sophomore year in college, I developed an anxiety disorder called obsessive-compulsive disorder or OCD. This OCD was coupled with depression (which I had throughout high school) and resulted in frequent insomnia throughout that year. I was still able to do well in school despite this, but I knew I had to do something about my comorbid insomnia. I sought counseling--which didn't help-- and I was also prescribed an anti-depressant called Prozac® which I couldn't tolerate.

Fortunately, during the second semester, I was taking a psychology course which covered the effectiveness of cognitive behavioral therapy or CBT for depression and anxiety. It soon occurred to me that CBT might also be effective for my chronic sleep problems. So, I did further research on it at the library and found an article in the American Journal of Psychiatry explaining how CBT was, in fact, an effective treatment for insomnia[13].

Eventually I implemented a self-help plan using CBT for overcoming my insomnia. Basically, I implemented most of the strategies found in this book. By the end of the semester, I found myself getting restful sleep almost every night! Furthermore, my anxiety and depression symptoms significantly improved because of it!

So, I personally experienced the health threat of chronic insomnia and how cognitive behavioral therapy for insomnia, or **CBT-I**, is a highly safe, tolerable, and effective treatment for overcoming insomnia.

Getting restful sleep through CBT-I will reap you many wonderful benefits. The quality of your life will greatly improve as you will feel more energetic, optimistic, and confident. With this newfound energy your relationships your relationships will improve and you will have the ability to set new you can set new goals that will bring even more meaning and happiness into your life! And, hopefully, you can lower your dependence upon sleeping pills or avoid them altogether!

How to Use This Book

The methods and strategies in this book are easy-to-understand and implement into your daily life. You will need to implement most of the strategies and techniques in this program. Although this book is for people who experience chronic sleep problems, it is also for those who want to prevent occasional insomnia from becoming chronic, and for those who just want to sleep better.

My CBT-I program is a 4-week program. On *day 1*, the first step is to read the introduction and Chapter 1-to learn the basic facts about sleep and CBT-I for insomnia. Next, you need to create and fill out a sleep diary for the first week or seven days to access your current baseline sleep pattern. You should continue to fill out a sleep diary for the entire four weeks so you can monitor your sleep pattern and the progress you are making. Finally, you should read Chapter 2 so that you can screen yourself for anxiety and depression.

This 4-week program consists of implementing four chapters.

Week	Chapter	Topic
One	Five	Cognitive Restructuring
Two	Three	Sleep Hygiene & Exercise
Three	Four	Using Behavioral Techniques
Four	Six	Reducing Your Stress Levels

In addition, in Chapter 4, you should choose the behavioral techniques that best suit you. However, you should use "Stimulus Control Therapy".

Although the self-help method is effective and worked for me, it has been proven that individual therapy or a face-to-face intervention with a therapist-for at least 4 sessions outperforms the self-help method[15]. Therefore, you might want to consider doing my CBT-I program with a therapist to further ensure your success. This is especially true if you are struggling with other issues such as anxiety and depression[16-17].

Chapter 1

Basic Facts about CBT-I for Insomnia

Cognitive-behavioral therapy for insomnia, or **CBT-I,** is an evidence-based treatment of insomnia that can be delivered in several formats: as individual therapy, group therapy, internet therapy and self-help therapy…in either its components or the full package[15]. Individual therapy (or face-to-face intervention with a therapist) is the most effective[15]. Nonetheless, self-help CBT-I is an increasingly popular treatment option for insomnia[18]. The robust results are similar for patients with or without comorbid disease, younger or older patients, using or not using sleep medication[15].

Sleep experts and primary care physicians consider this first-line treatment as the gold standard treatment for insomnia[19] because CBT-I treats the underlying causes of insomnia and does not have all the drawbacks of sleeping pills[20].

Currently, many patients are left untreated, as there is low reporting by patients, limited physician training in using CBT-I, and misconceptions about the seriousness of insomnia[21]. Because of this, our health organizations need to make sure that our primary physicians are aware of the safety and effectiveness of CBT-I when compared to medication and that they refer their insomnia patients over to a CBT-I program. Unfortunately, due to direct-to-consumer advertising, pharmaceutical companies have convinced the public of the safety and effectiveness of sleeping pills[22]. Pharmaceutical companies also exert significant control over the information that reaches physicians[23]. Consequently, sleep pharmacology is a huge industry.

The Superiority of CBT-I When Compared to Sleep Medication

Because CBT-I treats the underlying causes of insomnia

such as negative thoughts and cognitive distortions about sleep, it has lasting or permanent results[35]. In contrast, sleep medication only has short-term efficacy[35]. In addition, CBT-I has minimal side effects[36]. Furthermore, it is effective for comorbid insomnia[16,17,37].

CBT-I has even shown efficacy in patient populations that commonly have sleep problems and require medication. For example, in one study, patients with bipolar disorder overcame their insomnia by simply implementing *sleep hygiene*, s*timulus control therapy* and p*rogressive muscle relaxation* followed by strict regularity in bedtimes and rise times[38].

The most commonly prescribed drugs for insomnia are benzodiazepines such as Xanax® or alprazolam and nonbenzodiazepine hypnotics such as Ambien® or zolpidem. Although benzodiazepines (BZ's) such as Xanax are FDA approved for only short-term use (or up to 4 weeks) it is difficult to prevent short-term use from extending indefinitely[24]. The risks of BZ's are both physical and psychological[25]. In some patients, long-term use can lead to significant complications such as misuse, abuse, tolerance, dependence, and addiction[26-27]. Diagnosis of addiction (i.e. compulsive use despite negative consequences) may occur in vulnerable patients[26]. Because of this, BZ's are now recognized as major drugs of abuse and addiction[26]. In fact, in 2013 (as well as in previous years) Xanax was the number one selling psychiatric drug in America even though it was mainly used *off-label* for panic disorder and insomnia[28].

(Note: "Information in the National Prescription Audit (NPA) is derived from IMS Health's Xponent service, one of the most complete, national-level prescription databases in the U.S. Xponent captures roughly 70% Market Share of all prescriptions in the U.S. IMS then uses a patented projection methodology from a stratified and geographically balanced sample to represent 100% Market Share coverage of U.S. prescription activity at retail, mail service, long-term care, and managed care outlets[28]").

Patients should be advised of the potential negative side effects of BZ's such as cognitive dysfunction (i.e. anterograde amnesia)[29]; psychomotor impairment which includes the increased risk of falling in the elderly[30]. Finally, there is the risk of withdrawal syndrome[31]. Withdrawal syndrome or the physical and psychological side-effects from rapid or abrupt withdrawal from BZ use (such as rebound anxiety and seizures) can be stressful and dangerous[31]. Seizures usually occur if a patient has been taking a BZ for a long period of time and at a high dose. A gradual tapering off from a BZ is always necessary[31].

(Caution: **Never self-medicate or abruptly stop, change the dose, or taper off a benzodiazepine or any other drug without your doctor's approval; always follow your doctor's prescription and follow his or her guidelines for tapering off any drug**). In contrast to BZ's, nonbenzodiazepine hypnotics are only used for sleep or insomnia and are considered to be safer than BZ's[32]. However, these drugs, such as Ambien or zolpidem, do have abuse, addiction, and dependence capability[33]. Ambien® or zolpidem is the most widely prescribed nonbenzodiazepine hypnotic drug[34].

Sleep Diaries

When starting a CBT-I program you should access and record your current or baseline sleeping pattern on Day 1 for seven consecutive mornings. This should only take one minute of your time after you get out of bed. After seven consecutive mornings, you should be able to answer the following questions, in the following order, based on your sleep diaries:

- What time did you usually go to bed?

- How many nights did you have difficulty falling asleep?

- On these nights, how much time, on average, does it take you to fall asleep?

- How many nights per week do you wake up and have difficulty falling back asleep? On these nights, how many times did you typically wake up? How long did these awakenings last?

- On average, what is the total amount of time that you are awake during the night after these awakenings?

- How many days per week is your final wake-up earlier than desired?

- On nights when you have insomnia, how many hours, on average, do you sleep?

- On nights you don't have insomnia, how many hours, on average, do you sleep?

- How many nights per week do you take OTC (over the counter) or prescription sleeping pills? On these nights, what did you take and at what dose?

- What is your average sleep-quality rating on a scale of 1 to 5? (with 1 being very poor and 5 being very good).

Your answer to these questions represents your current sleep pattern, which will allow you to monitor your progress during this program. You should continue to fill out a sleep diary each morning throughout the four-week program. Completing the diary throughout this program is vital for tracking improvements in your sleep and supporting you in using the many techniques in this program. You should try to fit seven days into each sleep diary. Here is a sample.

Today's Date	11/02/20				
1. What time did you go to bed?	10:30 p.m.				
2. Did you have difficulty falling asleep?	No.				
3. How long did it take for you to fall asleep?	25 minutes				
4. Did you wake up before your final awakening and have difficulty falling back asleep? If so, how many times did you wake up? How long did these awakenings last?	Yes. Once. 1 hour.				
5. What time was your final awakening?	6:15 a.m.				
6. What time did you get out of bed?	6:30 a.m.				
7. In total, how many hours did you sleep?	6 hours.				
8. Did you take any OTC (over the counter) or sleep medication? If so, what did you take and at what dosage?	No.				

9.On a one to five scale, how would you rate the quality of your sleep? 1= very poor 2= poor 3= fair 4= good 5= very good	3				
10.Any additional comments?	I had a mild headache when I first went to bed.				

Using a Problem-Solving Log

Another useful exercise is to write down any problems or worries you typically have--at bedtime--*earlier in the day*. Simply write down your concerns and a plan of action. If your problem is overwhelming, you might want to discuss the problem with someone you know and trust. Writing or talking about these so-called problems or worries will at least ensure that you have a better perspective about them. When you get into bed you should be fully relaxed. If your troubles return as you doze off, tell yourself, "I've already worked that out."

Chapter 2

Ruling out Anxiety and Depression

By far, depression and anxiety are the most common psychiatric symptoms found in comorbid insomnia[39]. A study conducted by Dag Neckelmann, MD, PhD, of the Department of Psychiatry at Haukeland University Hospital in Bergen, Norway in 2007, was based on data collected from 25,130 adults from two general health surveys conducted over a 10-year period. Neckelmann found significant associations between the long-term course of chronic insomnia and the development of anxiety disorders and depression. "Chronic insomnia", says Neckelmann, "is a marker of both anxiety disorder and depression." says Neckelmann[39]. Furthermore, many people with depression and anxiety never seek treatment.

It's difficult to differentiate anxiety from depression because both anxious and depressed people experience distress, anger, fear, guilt, and worry[40,41]. However, only depressed individuals show the signs of fatigue and lack of energy and interest or enthusiasm, while people with anxiety experience symptoms of hyper-arousal which include a racing heart, trembling, dizziness, and shortness of breath[42].

In their helplessness/hopelessness model, Alloy and colleagues (1990) propose that anxiety and anxiety disorders are characterized by prominent feelings of helplessness[43]. People with these disorders expect that they may be helpless in controlling important outcomes, but they also believe that future control might be possible and so are likely to experience increased arousal and anxiety and an intense scanning of the environment in efforts to gain control.

If an individual becomes convinced of his helplessness to control important outcomes, but he is still uncertain about whether the bad outcome will occur, a mixed anxiety/depression syndrome is likely to emerge[43]. Finally, if an individual is also convinced that bad outcomes will occur, helplessness becomes hopelessness and depression will set in[43]. Thus, someone is likely to go through a stage of feeling helpless for some time before he or she feels the situation is hopeless.

This model makes perfect sense in the context of insomnia as it may be critical for you to get CBT treatment for insomnia as soon as possible to prevent the risk of developing depression. Our general practitioners need to be aware of this.

To help you determine whether you have an anxiety disorder or major depression, think about whether or not you have experienced any of the following symptoms on a consistent basis-or on most days-in the past 4 weeks.

1. Feeling so restless you can't sit still.

2. Feeling fearful.

3. Spells of terror or panic.

4. Feeling so nervous that nothing can calm you down.

5. Heart pounding or racing.

6. Feeling tired for no good reason.

7. Feeling hopeless about the future.

8. Loss of interest or pleasure in your normal daily activities.

9. Poor appetite.

10. Feeling so sad or blue that nothing can cheer you up.

11. Feeling worthless or guilty.

If you have experienced at least 2 of the symptoms of 1-5 you may have an anxiety disorder, and if you have experienced at least 3 of the symptoms of 6-11, you may have major depression. If you suspect you have an anxiety disorder and/or major depression you should seek professional evaluation and treatment.

Fortunately, CBT-I has also been proven to alleviate anxiety and depression as you overcome your sleep problems. This is especially true with individual therapy[16,18].

If better sleep does not alleviate your anxiety and depressive symptoms, it might be wise to see a therapist or get some relief from an anti-depressant drug such as an SSRI. In monotherapy, SSRI's (anti-depressants such as Zoloft® (sertraline) and

Lexapro® (escitalopram)) are considered first-line treatment for major depression as they are effective, safe, and tolerable[44]. Furthermore, SSRI's treat OCD and other types of anxiety disorders. Your doctor can help you find the one that is most suitable for your individual needs. And, if you so desire, you can safely taper off an anti-depressant drug. **Be sure to strictly follow your doctor's guidelines whenever you taper off any medication.**

The best nondrug treatment for anxiety and depression is cognitive therapy. Cognitive therapy is based on the premise that our negative moods come from our negative, distorted thoughts.

As with any disease, the sooner you get treatment for anxiety and depression, the better off you will be.

Chapter 3

Sleep Hygiene

The goal of sleep hygiene is to separate sleep from wakefulness.

1. As soon as possible, restrict yourself to your ideal bedtime and rise time every day, including weekends. This is probably the most important step in Sleep Hygiene because in itself, it can ensure restful sleep. It is also important because regular exposure to light in the morning is what sets the brain's alarm clock. This exposure will establish the time to wake up and, at night, the time to get drowsy again.

2. If you are short on sleep because of insomnia, do not simply go to bed earlier. This only results in longer periods of lousy sleep. Instead, decrease your sleep time by retiring later--when you are genuinely sleepy--and rising earlier. You may end up getting less rest, but you know you will sleep soundly, so you will lose your apprehension about it.

3. Get aerobic exercise on a regular basis (such as walking or speed walking, hiking, swimming, bike riding and cross-country skiing). You should exercise preferably every day or at least every other day and for at least 30 minutes.

If you can't get exercise outdoors you should use a treadmill or an elliptical at home or at a gym. It's healthiest to get your exercise under the sun and earlier in the day (see section on "Exercise"). Do not exercise within 4 hours of bedtime.

4. Make sure to eat plenty of fruits and vegetables on a regular basis for energy and to avoid large meals close to bedtime. I enjoy eating apples, bananas, and carrots on a regular basis.

5. Reserve caffeine for earlier in the day. Avoid energy drinks. Avoid a lot of sugar close to bedtime (especially if you are diabetic). Avoid nicotine and alcohol close to bedtime. There should be at least a 3-hour separation between alcohol and sleep. Regular alcohol consumption

should be restricted to one drink for women and two drinks for men.

6. Talk to your doctor before using any new supplement. Many supplements can disturb your sleep pattern or cause insomnia. Remember that supplements are not FDA regulated and can be just as dangerous as prescription drugs.

7. If possible, you should avoid taking any naps during the day. If it is necessary to take a nap, restrict it to 30 minutes. This rule helps you maintain your regular sleep-wake cycle.

8. Keep your bedroom light off throughout the day and turn off as many lights as you can at dusk[48].

9. Avoid using an electronic device within three hours of bedtime. If using an Ipad or PC near bedtime is inevitable, download "justgetflux.com" software on to your electronic device for free. f.lux® makes the color of your computer's display adapt to the time of day, warm at night and like sunlight during the day.

10. Do not avoid or cancel social or family obligations when you don't get enough sleep. Being fully active during the day helps to ensure restful sleep.

11. Reserve your bedroom for only intimacy and sleep.

Exercise

Exercise is an important component for treating insomnia because it uplifts your mood, effectively reduces your stress levels, and helps you feel sleepier at the end of the day[45]. According to Charlene Gamaldo, M.D., medical director of John Hopkins Center for Sleep, "We have solid evidence that exercise does, in fact, help you fall asleep more quickly and improves sleep quality[66]." According to the National Sleep Foundation's 2013 *Sleep in America*® poll, "Vigorous exercisers are almost twice as likely as non-exercisers to report "I had a good night's sleep" every night or almost every night during the week[46]."

From personal experience, I know that **speed walking** (which is vigorous exercise) for at least 30 minutes five days a week had an immediate effect on alleviating my stress, improving my mood, and inducing restful sleep so I can stay on a regular schedule.

So, if you want to further ensure restful sleep, I highly recommend vigorous aerobic exercise such as speed walking, jogging, hiking, cross-country skiing, or swimming for at least 30 minutes and up to an hour…especially earlier in the day.

It is well known that regular exercise is very good for the brain and can also prevent type 2 diabetes[47]. Furthermore, vigorous exercise will give you energy for the rest of the day. In fact, it is even effective for treating chronic fatigue syndrome[48].

Finally, exercise not only keeps the heart healthy and get oxygen into the system, but it helps deplete stress hormones and releases mood-enhancing chemicals, such as endorphins, which help us cope better with stress. **Endorphins** are often classified as the "happy hormones". Any form of physical activity leads to the release of these "feel good" neurotransmitters. The increase in endorphins in your body leads to a feeling of euphoria, modulation of your appetite, and enhances your immune system.

Professor Marco Mello, an NSF sleep poll task force member, adds: "In addition to exercise, standing at your desk, getting up for short breaks, and moving around as much as possible are important healthy behaviors to include in our lives[46]."

Unfortunately, restful sleep doesn't necessarily motivate us to exercise. But the benefit of just feeling better makes exercise a wonderful practice. The famous philosopher Soren Kierkegaard once wrote to his niece: "Above all, do not lose our desire to walk. Every day I walk myself into a state of well-being and walk away from every illness. I have walked into my best thoughts, and I know of no thought so burdensome that one cannot walk away from it...thus, if one just keeps on walking, everything will be alright[49]."

Even a short walk every day is beneficial. According to Max Hirshkowitz, PhD., another NSF sleep poll task force member,

"If you are inactive, adding a ten-minute walk everyday can improve your likelihood of a good night's sleep[46]."

Chapter 4

Behavioral Therapy

Stimulus Control Therapy

The purpose of this type of behavioral therapy is to re-establish the connection between the bed and sleep. Your goal is to associate your bed with drowsiness.

1. Go to bed only when drowsy.

2. Use the bed and bedroom only for sleep and intimacy.

3. Avoid trying to force sleep. If you cannot fall asleep within 25 minutes when you first go to bed, be sure to get out of your bed and leave the room. When you are up, do something that is relaxing such as watching television or reading a book. Go back to bed only when you feel drowsy. Repeat this process as often as necessary until you fall asleep.

4. Do not watch the clock whether you are in or out of bed.

5. Do not worry, plan, or problem-solve in bed. Just relax and enjoy the peace and comfort of being in bed and falling asleep.

Sleep Deprivation Method

People with chronic insomnia often display widely varying times of retiring and rising from bed, with consequent variability in the timing of light exposure, social interaction, physical activity, and other stimuli that dictate their circadian system.

The *sleep deprivation method* is a popular and effective strategy for resetting your body for your ideal bedtime and rising time or your sleep-wake cycle. A good target range for sleep deprivation is 28 to 36 hours. To get through a sleep deprivation period try to do things you really enjoy doing such as watching a favorite movie, listening to music and reading. And do not play video games on the second night.

For example, if you work Monday through Friday, you

should get up on Saturday at the same time you do on a workday and stay up all Saturday night and stay up all Sunday (without taking any naps) and go to bed Sunday night at a time which allows you to get your optimal level of sleep for Monday morning. Most people only require 8 hours of sleep, but it does vary among individuals.

By using the *sleep deprivation method,* you can be rest assured that your sleep problem will be solved and there will be no need for worrying about falling asleep on the last night. After using this method, be sure to restrict yourself to your ideal bedtime and rising time even on days that you want to sleep in.

Progressive Relaxation

Relaxation practices help bring the body back into balance and regulate the flight-or-response we feel when we are stressed. This is particularly helpful if you are experiencing sleeplessness due to anxiety or worries about what happened today--or what might happen tomorrow.

Progressive muscle relaxation (PMR) is a relaxation therapy which was first developed by Chicago physician Edmund Jacobson, MD, in 1915 and was published in the 1920's. PMR is a relaxation exercise in which you systematically tense and then relax all the muscle groups of your body. It was based on the premise that mental calmness is the natural result of physical relaxation.

In addition to helping you fall asleep, PMR promotes a better sense of overall well-being, can lower your blood pressure, reduces muscle tension, and reduces anxiety. PMR can be learned by nearly anyone and requires only 10 to 20 minutes per day to practice and then use it just before going to bed or after getting into bed.

Most practitioners recommend tensing and relaxing the different muscle groups one at a time in a specific order, generally beginning with the lower extremities and ending with the face, abdomen, and chest. You can practice this technique seated or lying down, and you should try to practice with comfortable clothing on, and in a quiet place free of all distractions.

First, while inhaling, contract one muscle group for 5 seconds, then exhale and suddenly release the tension in that muscle group. While releasing the tension, try to focus on the changes you feel when the muscle group is relaxed. Next, give yourself 10 to 20 seconds to relax and then move on to the next muscle group. Starting with your legs and feet, gradually work your way up the body.

- **Legs and feet.** Using the guideline above, curl your toes for 5 to 10 seconds and then relax them.
  Next, flex your calf muscles and relax them. Finally, flex your thigh muscles and relax them.
- **Buttocks.** Tighten the muscles in your buttocks and then release the tension.

- **Back.** Flex the muscles in your back as you arch them on the floor, couch, or bed, and then relax and let the tension go out of your back muscles.

- **Shoulders and arms.** Tense your shoulders by moving them in a circular motion for 5 to 10 seconds and then relax them. Next, place your hands on your hips and tense your biceps and then relax them.

- **Face.** Lift your eyebrow to wrinkle your forehead and then slowly relax and let the tension leave your forehead. Close your eyes tightly and then relax and slowly open them. Tense your lips, cheeks, and jaw muscles by grimacing, and then feel a sense of serenity come over your face as you relax all your facial muscles at once.

- **Abdomen.** Take a deep breath and tense the muscles in your abdomen and then release the tension.

- **Chest.** Take a deep breath and tense the muscles in your chest and then release the tension.

Breathing Techniques

Breathing techniques, like progressive muscle relaxation, helps calm your mind and distracts you from racing thoughts. There are three breathing techniques that I highly recommend. The first one I will cover, which I use, is the 4-7-8 breathing technique.

4-7-8 Breathing Technique

Dr. Andrew Weil developed this technique as a variation of *pranayama*, an ancient yogic technique that helps people relax as it replenishes oxygen in the body. Dr. Weil has even described it as a natural tranquilizer for the nervous system[59]."

Here is how to practice the 4-7-8 breathing technique:

1. Allow your lips to gently part.
2. Exhale completely, making a breathy *whoosh* sound as you do.

3. Press your lips together as you silently inhale through the nose for a count of 4 seconds.

4. Hold your breath for a count of 7 seconds.

5. Exhale again for a full 8 seconds, making a whooshing sound throughout.

Repeat 4 times when you first start. Eventually work up to 8 repetitions.

Three-part Breathing Exercise

Some people prefer this technique over others because of its sheer simplicity[59].

To practice the three-part breathing exercise, follow these three steps:

1. Take a long, deep inhale.

2. Exhale fully while focusing intently on your body and how it feels.

After doing this a few times, slow down your exhale so that it is twice as long as your inhale.

Buteyko Breathing

Many people do not realize that they are hyper-ventilating. This technique helps you to reset to a normal breathing rhythm[59].

1. Sit in bed with your mouth gently closed (not pursed) and breathe through your nose at a natural pace for about 30 seconds.

2. Breathe a bit more intentionally in and out through your nose once.

3. Gently pinch your nose closed with your thumb and forefinger, keeping your mouth closed as well, until you feel that you need to take a breath again.

With your mouth still closed, take a deep breath in and out through your nose again.

Visualization

Visualization can be a powerful technique to help you unwind, relieve stress, and even fall asleep. It is also short and simple. Instead of focusing on your anxious, fearful images, visualization expands your ability to focus on calming and restful images. While everyone can visualize, some people can visualize much deeper and more vividly than others. Those who can visualize much deeper are the ones that will truly benefit from this technique.

The first step is to get into a comfortable position in bed, then close your eyes and relax. Next, begin to visualize a scene where you feel deeply relaxed and peaceful. It may be on a beach, in a kayak, or in the woods on a sunny day. Try to notice any details in these images and focus upon them. This technique should only take five to ten minutes.

Paradoxical Intention

This technique is effective for those with acute or intense performance anxiety about falling asleep or falling back asleep. You are supposed to intentionally engage in your most feared behavior (usually staying relaxed and awake without any worries about sleep or being completely detached about falling asleep). First off, you have to let your mind run freely and divert your attention to whatever is going on inside yourself. Next, fully accept the state that you are in or your life situation. Pay full attention to the present moment and to your breathing. Feel the power of your presence and narrow your life down to this moment. Finally, create some space, so that you find the life underneath your life situation.

I once used paradoxical intention successfully without even knowing it. I had a stressful day and I decided to go to bed early knowing that I had a poor chance of falling asleep. It was early in the evening and I could hear kids playing outside of my house.

Anyway, I decided that I was just going to relax as much as possible in bed without even thinking about whether or not I was going to fall asleep. But something else was going on too. I was totally accepting of my "life situation" and I became deeply rooted within my body and was focused only on the present moment. I could fully feel the power of my presence and find the life underneath my life situation.

The best way to describe this process is that *mentally* I "died while being alive" (I've come across this concept in different books). I was feeling the power of my own presence…which is to say I was connected with my "Being" and felt the joy of just "Being". In other words, instead of feeling any anxiety, I was fully enjoying being awake in bed and being in the present moment. Anyway, this whole "process" took about 45 minutes and then I fell asleep and stayed asleep for nine hours.

Fortunately, I now know the exact "process" that I went through simply because I read a book called "Practicing the Power of Now" by Eckhart Tolle which I highly recommend reading and using. Some of the terminology that I used above comes from his book. According to Tolle, "When you are present, when your attention is fully and intensely in the Now, "Being" can be felt, but it can never be understood mentally.[67]" Therefore, "Paradoxical Intention" is a form of mindfulness-based cognitive therapy in which you find your deepest self or your true nature.

Inherent in this exercise, however, is that you do not pay any attention to how much time you spend in bed. Some people may find this to be anxiety provoking but it certainly doesn't have to be.

Chapter 5

Cognitive Therapy

Two of the earliest forms of Cognitive Behavioral Therapy are Rational Emotive Behavior Therapy (REBT), developed by Albert Ellis in the 1950's, and Cognitive Therapy, developed by Aaron T. Beck in the 1960's. CBT was found to be very effective for major depression. CBT is now used for many problems. The basic premise of cognitive therapy is that *the way we think has a strong influence on the way we feel, and therefore changing how we think can change the way we feel.*

Many people report an increase in anxiety when they are unable to fall asleep and upon further assessment, it is evident that the content of their thoughts is what causes it. Besides causing anxiety and frustration, negative sleep thoughts increase your heart rate, blood pressure, muscle tension, and breathing rate…all of which speed up your brain waves causing you to be awake. Most people with insomnia repeat in their minds negative statements concerning sleep and insomnia.

Cognitive therapy for insomnia, also known as **cognitive restructuring,** is very powerful because it teaches us to identify negative thoughts and beliefs about sleep and insomnia and replace them with more rational and accurate ones. Clients are encouraged to remain in bed, relax their body, and most importantly, make a mental shift to more positive thoughts. Eventually, you will have a new frame of reference or way to view sleep and insomnia.

Tonight, when in bed, reflect on any of your automatic thoughts and identify the negative ones. As soon as you do, think of a more positive and accurate thought to replace the negative one. For example, you might think *"If I don't get enough sleep, people are going to notice that I'm not as productive at work tomorrow"* and replace that thought with

"I don't have to get a full eight hours of sleep to be fully productive at work tomorrow...four or five hours will be enough." The very next day you should **write down** every negative thought that you are aware of and then write down a replacement thought.

Here is a list of accurate and positive thoughts about sleep and insomnia:

- Bedtime is always a good time to just relax.
- Falling asleep is relaxing.
- Falling asleep is effortless bliss.
- It is easy to relax and stay relaxed in bed when I use the techniques in this program.
- I may not sleep well now as I am new to this CBT-I program, but my sleep will get better as I continue treatment.
- It is perfectly normal to have an occasional sleepless night.
- It is wrong to think people will notice that I am incompetent at work when I don't get enough sleep. Most people with occasional insomnia function quite well.

- Occasional sleeplessness is not going to cause me any health problems because the human body is resilient with maintaining adequate mental and physical health.

- Since I didn't sleep well last night, I am much more likely to sleep well tonight.

- Falling back asleep is just as easy as falling asleep the first time.

- I will always fall asleep sleep sooner or later.

- Cognitive-behavioral therapy for insomnia has an 80 percent success rate[36].

Cognitive Distortions

Cognitive distortions are thinking errors people have when they feel afraid or anxious. The following list contains some cognitive distortions that people with insomnia often fall victim to.

1. Catastrophizing occurs when people focus on the worst possible outcome when they have sleep problems. A person with insomnia might think, "If I don't get enough sleep, I won't be as productive at work and I will probably get fired." This is faulty thinking because you will still be productive enough at work even if you do not get enough sleep.

2. All-or-nothing thinking occurs when an individual decides that he or she will never overcome their sleep problems. This can lead to feelings of hopelessness and depression. In reality, CBT-I is a viable sleep solution for 80 percent of all users.

3. Emotional Reasoning occurs when an individual lets his or her feelings guide their interpretation of reality rather than the facts. For example, a worry-prone individual being even more convinced that she will not get enough sleep because she feels anxious or more anxious than usual about falling asleep. Or an individual might feel anxiety during the evening and will conclude that they probably won't be able to fall asleep at bedtime even though they know that the anxiety will probably be gone by bedtime.

Depressed people commonly end up reasoning emotionally. They may engage in filtering and focus on one piece of bad news in a set of mostly positive news, and then decide that the bad news means that things are hopeless. It does not matter if they actually have the power to influence their situation, because this will be overlooked if emotional reasoning holds its ground.

And it's not just depressed people who reason emotionally. Almost everyone does this sort of thing on a regular basis. People like to think that they are usually logical decision-makers, but unfortunately, this is not generally the case. The human brain simply has a tendency to make a decision based on feeling rather than on facts. We tend to not look at all the facts to support our conclusions; we just accept a conclusion because it feels right.

4. Jumping to conclusions occurs when an individual expects that sleeplessness is likely to occur based on poor evidence. The *truth* is that you should expect and look forward to getting restful sleep when you use the techniques in this program. Another example would be when an individual decides that CBT-I will not work after implementing only one strategy such as *sleep hygiene*.

Once you can identify a cognitive distortion, you can replace it with a more rational and positive thought.

A big misconception is that falling asleep is something that we *try* to accomplish. However, falling asleep is not something you *try* to do, it is something you just *do*. Just as birds don't try to fly, they just fly. In other words, falling asleep is supposed to be effortless because it is a natural process of the brain.

Whatever progress you have made with cognitive restructuring, you still need to accept your current level of consciousness when you get into bed. By this, I mean you still need to fully accept whatever negative thoughts that still occupy your mind, because cognitive restructuring is a gradual process. When you get into bed, *let your mind run freely; do not resist any racing thoughts; be in the present moment.* Of course, being in the present moment is the best way to live your life as well. Just look at children; they live in the present moment all day long--happy and carefree--and when they go to bed at night they sleep like babies!

If you regularly find yourself stuck in a negative mind-set when you go to bed, I highly recommend practicing "Mindfulness Meditation" (next chapter) in the evening or before bedtime. You will find yourself in a much more relaxed and positive state of mind when you go to bed.

An important goal of cognitive therapy is that instead of viewing sleep as something you *have* to do, you begin to view sleep as something you *get* to do. You look forward to going to bed and enjoy the entire process of sleep.

Chapter 6

Reducing Your Stress Levels

Stress can be both the cause and result of insomnia. Keeping stress at a minimal level throughout the day can ensure restful sleep. Unfortunately, too many people today create unnecessary stress in their lives due to conflicting values, negative attitudes, poor time management, an unhealthy lifestyle, and inertia. Uncontrolled stress easily leads to anxiety and depression as well. It produces the hormone *cortisol*, which is highly associated with weight gain. By reducing or preventing stress in our lives, we are literally protecting our physical and psychological well-being.

The biggest cause of stress is a negative attitude towards life, other people, and oneself. A negative attitude stems from our consistent and unchallenged automatic negative thoughts which are the result of our expectations and our beliefs about "what is" and "what will be" or our life-situation. These beliefs can easily become a self-fulfilling prophecy so that "as we think, we will experience."

For example, if you have the distorted belief that, "People are not trustworthy"-you will have a very difficult time finding and building new and healthy relationships which we need to maintain a healthy or positive attitude. In contrast, the general and rational belief that people are good and trustworthy will lead to the opportunity of building new and healthy relationships and you will experience positive emotions. Another empowering belief might be, "I strongly prefer life to be fair, easy and hassle-free and it's very frustrating that it isn't, but I can bear frustration and still considerably enjoy life."

According to Tolle, "Almost everyone, in varying degrees, suffers from the mind-identified state[67]." But you should know that you *are not* your thoughts; rather, you *are* the thinker or observer behind your thoughts.

Healthy people are not overly attached to their problems as they have good coping skills. They resist becoming negative, bitter, or hopeless in times of struggle. They are not easily provoked into anger and they make the best out of any current situation. They can easily forgive and forget. They have love and compassion for themselves as well as for others. Finally, they live in the present and are less controlled by their egos which try to convince them that they need to be in control, to be approved, and to judge.

Positive Illusions

Positive thoughts can promote what is called **positive illusions** which are a collection of stress reducing thoughts and beliefs. In daily life, many situations are ambiguous and can be perceived in many different ways. Moreover, since we all distort reality through our individual mental filters anyway (such as our thoughts and belief system), we should choose to create a reality which improves the quality of our lives. Hence, the term "reality" is a contradiction in terms because there is no actual reality, only the perception of it.

I came across the concept of "positive illusions" while reading about CBT in a psychology textbook. Dr. Shelley Taylor, and her colleague Jonathan Brown (1988), published an article "Illusion and Well-being: A Social Psychological Perspective on Mental Health"[50] and it was based on hundreds of individual experiences. I searched for information on this article through the internet, and I came across an article in the New York Times titled "Mental Health; Trying to Face Reality? It May Be the Last Thing That the Doctor Orders" by Daniel Goldman[51]. The article was a summary based on Dr. Taylor's work and I found it to be remarkable.

Here is the summary: "Psychologists have found that stress-resistant people are more than just optimistic: they distort reality in order to view it in the best possible light. A bit of illusion, of clinging to false hopes and inflated self-regard, may be the bedrock of psychological health, according to evidence emerging from a broad range of scientific studies. Certain positive illusions, the data suggest, promote a sense of well-being and happiness and the capacity for productive work.

The evidence seriously questions the belief that facing reality is a hallmark of mental health. Instead, it suggests that, within limits, living a life of illusion is normal and healthy. The "healthy" illusions include an unrealistically positive view of oneself, an exaggerated sense of control and an unfounded optimism.

To be sure, there are limits to how far one can cling to illusion. The old clinical wisdom that reality (no matter how bitter) was needed for mental health is based to a large extent on work with people who were grossly out of touch. For *such* people, Dr. Taylor acknowledges, stronger contact with reality is needed.

However, for the majority of people, who do not suffer a severe mental disorder, "there is a more moderate range of illusion that seems to be essential to their sense of stability", she argues. "Such illusions put a kind of positive twist on information about yourself," Dr. Taylor said. "Negative facts are not experienced as so negative, and positive ones are experienced as even more positive."

"People negotiate their days by drawing strength from positive illusions," says Dr. Taylor. "If you woke up knowing in advance how little you'd accomplish, about the awful times you'd have with people, about the rejections you'd get, why would you even get out of bed? Positive illusions spawn optimism." Positive illusions such as these, Dr. Taylor believes, also help people overcome devastating events such as a cancer patient who has a recurrence of tumors[51].

Several researchers have found, for instance, that as people become mildly depressed, they begin to become more candid in their view of themselves, seeing the flaws more clearly." However, according to Dr. Richard Lazarus from the University of California at Berkley, "Mildly depressed people are very realistic about themselves, in fact, *too* realistic[51]".

"Friends and family also join individuals in a tacit conspiracy to perpetuate positive illusions", Dr. Taylor said. Research suggests that may be "one reason that supportive social contacts are associated with better physical and emotional health" (see next section). Dr. Taylor was careful to point out that not just any illusion is helpful. "Some illusions are adaptive, others are not," adding that "any illusions should not be completely warped to be healthy, but mildly distorted in a positive direction[51]."

An example of a "positive illusion" that I use in my personal life is the phrase, "Don't sweat the small stuff...and it's all small stuff" which is the title of a best-selling book by the late author Richard Carlson. What matters most in life is not what happens, but how you respond to what happens. The poet John Milton once wrote: "The mind is its own place and in itself, can make a Heaven of Hell, a Hell of Heaven."

Social Support

Social support is exceptionally important for maintaining good physical and mental health. Overall, it appears that positive social support of high quality can enhance resilience to stress, help protect against developing trauma-related psycho-pathology, decrease the functional consequences of trauma-induced disorders, such as posttraumatic stress disorder (PTSD), and reduce medical morbidity and mortality[52]. The effect of social support on life expectancy appears to be as strong as the effects of obesity, cigarette smoking, hypertension, or your level of physical activity.

The positive emotions resulting from social support-such as love, contentment, and warmth--reduce stress and its symptoms. Social support also plays a part in protecting or supporting our brain function as we age. Social support also exerts positive effects on health because it allows us to: share feelings and receive helpful suggestions, seek solutions to problems, reframe negative thoughts and change behavior, develop a sense of reliability and stability in times of transition, shift attention away from ourselves to something larger.

Unfortunately, the conditions of modern life have led to an increase in social isolation and lack of connectedness. Throughout evolution, man lived in extended kin networks, surrounded by genetic relatives such as aunts and uncles, nephews and nieces. But in the past several decades, social ties have been disrupted by mobility, fragmentation of the nuclear and extended family, single-parent families, and separations and divorces. Few of us have parents who live nearby, and few enjoy the same close-knit communities that existed in previous generations. Life-long friendships are not as common. Most of us do not just drop over to a friend's house unannounced as was the case years ago. As a population, we are more likely to live alone, remain unmarried, and far less likely to belong to a social organization. One of the great ironies of modern life may

be that, despite being surrounded by many more people than
our distant ancestors were, we have fewer intimate
relationships and more loneliness and isolation than any other
time period in human history.

Religious and Spiritual Beliefs

Although religion and science have been kept separate in
modern times, and often seem at odds, there have been over a
dozen studies confirming that religion reduces stress and
improves our mental health[53]. In fact, any kind of religious belief
can be a powerful way of coping with adversity[54]. The most
popular religion in America today is Christianity, comprising the
majority of the adult population at 73.7 percent[60].

Based on personal experience, as a Christian, I personally
believe in a God who is both all-powerful and all good, and who
has given us the gift of free will. Unfortunately, free will can be
used for evil. I also believe it is our duty to always forgive those

who have trespassed against us…and that to truly forgive you need to both forgive and *forget*.

In his popular book, "The Purpose Driven Life", author Rick Warren states: "You cannot arrive at your life's purpose by starting with a focus on yourself. You must begin with God, your Creator. You exist only because God wills that you exist. You were made *by* God and *for* God--and until you understand that, life will never make sense[68]." God *is* love and "it is only in Him that we discover our origin, our identity, our meaning, our purpose, our significance, and out destiny. Every other path leads to a dead end[68]."

Although having the Christian faith is definitely rewarding, being a true Christian is not an easy path to take in today's world. *Materialism,* for example, can be a major obstacle. The root of materialism is the belief that we need to get what we want when we want in order to be happy. In contrast, Jesus said "Do not worry about having enough" (Matt. 6:25 ESV) and to "Seek the kingdom of God above all else, and live righteously, and he will give you everything you need" (Matt. 6:33 NLT) and "to be in the world, but not of the world" (John 15:19, 17:14 NKJV). Money and pleasure can never give you real joy or happiness. You can only experience real joy if God is within you.

One of the greatest attributes of being Christian is our belief in an afterlife or Heaven, which gives us the virtue of hope as well as a strong sense of purpose and meaning. For in Scripture, it is written: What no eye has seen, nor ear heard, nor the heart of man imagined, what God has prepared for those who love Him" (1 Cor 2:9 ESV). Outside of the Bible, there have been books about near death experiences that strongly support the existence of Heaven such as "Heaven is for Real" by Todd Burpo and "90 Minutes in Heaven: A true Story of Death and Life" by Don Piper.

Mel Gibson is an excellent example of someone who found the value of having the Christian faith. After all of his material success, he realized that something was missing. "He looked at the Oscars, the money, all that fame and fortune, and decided there had to be more[78]." He eventually produced and directed the successful film "The Passion of the Christ" in 2004.

In addition, a book called "Jesus Calling" (2004) by Sarah Young has been a major success. There have been well over 10 million copies sold and it has reached to #1 on the Wall Street Journal's Non-Fiction Bestseller list. Each year 'Jesus Calling' sells more books than the year before[64]. I believe that there has been somewhat of a "spiritual revival" going on in America today…indicating that we are ready to believe. If you want to learn more about the truth of Christianity, I highly recommend reading "Mere Christianity" which is an apologetic book written by C.S. Lewis.

Meditation for Reducing Stress

While too much stress can easily lead to occasional insomnia, meditation induces restful sleep by slowing down your brain

waves and thereby reducing your stress levels[55]. In addition to
improving sleep, it has been proven that meditation reduces high
blood pressure, pain, acute respiratory illnesses, and that it
improves your digestive and immune system as well as supports
your cognition[55].

Officially, there are six types of meditation: Mindfulness
Meditation, Spiritual Meditation (such as Christian
Meditation), Focused Meditation, Moment Meditation, Mantra
Meditation, and Transcendental Meditation®[56]. I will cover the
two which I practice: Christian Meditation and Mindfulness
Meditation.

Christian Meditation

Christian Meditation is a form of spiritual meditation that is
both uplifting and effective in reducing your stress levels. Of
course, using Christian Meditation is a personal choice.
Christians of various traditions still encourage meditation as a
means to get closer to God. Eastern-style meditation, in contrast,

generally involves "emptying the mind." *Biblical contemplation* and *prayer* are the two forms of Christian Meditation.

Biblical contemplation is about reflecting upon the meaning of Scripture or "God's Word" with the goal of strengthening our hearts and minds with confidence and faith and producing faith-filled thoughts and actions. I personally use biblical contemplation because it strengthens and encourages me on a regular basis. In his book, "The Power of Positive Thinking", Dr. Norman Vincent Peale urges us to "drop the words of the Bible into your mind, allowing them to "dissolve" in consciousness, as they spread a healing balm over your entire mental structure[62]. Reflecting upon the meaning of Scripture is a powerful way to attain a healthy and strong positive attitude. I first read "The Power of Positive Thinking" when I was a teenager and through the years two biblical passages from that book have always stuck with me: "I can do all things through Christ, who strengthens me" (Philippians 4:13 NKJV) and "If God be for us, who can be against us?" (Romans 8:31 NIV). Both of these biblical passages uplift the human soul.

In addition to "The Power of Positive Thinking", there are many other successful spiritual growth books that are also filled with powerful, uplifting Scripture, such as "The Purpose Driven Life" by Rick Warren, "Fearless" by Max Lucado, "God Calling" by A.J. Russell, and "No Man Is an Island" by Thomas Merton.

I know from personal experience that when your life hits rock bottom the only thing that can really set you free is reading and meditating upon Scripture--for at least a good hour. It is the only option you can truly depend on.

I highly recommend that you spend at least 20 minutes every day, or on a regular basis, reflecting upon powerful Scripture to pour-in God's truth. Some people prefer doing this in the morning while others prefer doing it in the evening or near bedtime.

Most of my personal biblical contemplation is practiced through the Book of Psalms and the Book of Proverbs (both of them are Wisdom Books) as well the entire New Testament. A popular biblical verse among Christians is found in Psalm 23:

"The Lord is my shepherd, I lack nothing.

He makes me to lie down in green pastures, he leads me beside quiet waters,

he refreshes my soul. He guides me along the right paths for his name's sake.

Even though I walk through the darkest valley,

I will fear no evil,

for you are with me; your rod and your staff comfort me.

You prepare a table before me in the presence of my enemies.

You anoint my head with oil; my cup overflows.

Surely your goodness and love will follow me all the days of my life, and I will dwell in the house of the Lord Forever" (Psalm 23:1-6 NIV).

In Psalm 37:4 it is written: "Take delight in the Lord and you will be given the desires of your heart" (NIV). Of course, to "Take delight in the Lord" means following in the steps of Jesus. Jesus had only two major commandments: To love God and to love your neighbor as yourself.

Another favorite of mine is "Be still and know that I am God" (Psalm 46:10 NIV). To me, this verse is telling us to be in the present moment, to just "relax", to "let go" and to "cease striving". This passage relates directly to a wonderful quote by Mother Teresa (Anjeze Gonxhe Bojaxhiu) (1910-1997): "Be happy in the moment, that's enough. Each moment is all we need, not more."

Outside of the Bible, you can also meditate upon the famous Serenity Prayer by American theologian Reinhold Niebuhr: "God give me the grace to accept with serenity

the things that cannot be changed, Courage to

change the things which should be changed, and

the Wisdom to distinguish the one from the other.

Living one day at a time,

Enjoying one moment at a time,

Accepting hardship as a pathway to peace,

Taking, as Jesus did,

This sinful world as it is,

Not as I would have it,

Trusting that You will make all things right,

If I surrender to Your will,

So that I may be reasonably happy in this life, And

supremely happy with You forever in the next.

Amen.

The second component of Christian Meditation is **prayer**. It has been known for a long time that praying for others (even for complete strangers) has been scientifically proven to have a healing effect[63]. You have the choice of using either short prayer or deep prayer. Personally, I tend to use short prayer more frequently than deep prayer. Most nights, when I get into bed, I will say the Lord's Prayer, which is also called the Our Father prayer, as well as the Hail Mary prayer. Deep prayer, on the other hand, is much more time-consuming, but has even a stronger effect on slowing down your brain waves because you are connecting more with God.

Making direct contact with God through deep prayer is a purely natural process in which you can relax and just be yourself. You can thank God for all the things he has blessed you with..."for everything good comes from him" (James 1:17). Furthermore, sincere gratitude begets happiness.

With deep prayer, people sometimes think that they are praying wrong simply because they don't feel anything. But this is only how it seems to be. Soon enough, you will discover that God, through his Spirit, will respond to your conscious thinking or "groaning" and you will experience a "peace that surpasses all understanding" (Phil. 4:7 ESV). You will find yourself outside of space and time.

You should never doubt the power of God. For when we trust in him we receive his divine mercy. The prophet Isaiah proclaimed: "You will keep him in perfect peace, whose mind is stayed on You, because he trusts in You" (Isaiah 26:3 ESV). Furthermore, in Matthew, it is written, "Ask and it will be given to you" (Matthew 7:7 NIV). For there is nothing we cannot ask for and receive if it increases our love for God or his love for us. You should try to be specific in what you ask for. I believe, as did Dr. Norman Vincent Peale, that any negative habit can be changed with the help of God.

God wants us to shape our own destiny in the way he has planned it for us. In Jeremiah, the LORD declares, "For I know the plans I have for you; plans to prosper you and not harm you, plans to give you a hope and a future" (Jeremiah 29:11 NIV). Through Jesus Christ, God promises forgiveness and helps us to overcome the temptations and weaknesses that reside in all of us. All he asks of us is to seek holiness and righteousness and to have a personal relationship with him. Remember that "God has not given us a spirit of fear, but a spirit of power, and of love, and of sound mind" (2 Timothy 1:7 NKJV).

Mindfulness Meditation

Mindfulness Meditation is a simple but powerful form of meditation, which I use whenever I find myself stuck in a negative mindset or emotion. I have successfully used Mindfulness Meditation many times. It comprises of getting rid of a negative emotion by simply focusing on any tension in your body--specifically your stomach and chest. You should simply sit or lay down (I prefer laying down), close your eyes, remain calm, and focus exclusively on the tension or sensations in your body for at least 20 minutes. Tension in your upper chest, for example, indicates a feeling of anxiety or fear. Remember to breathe freely as there is no special way to breathe while doing this meditation technique although it is fine to be aware of your breathing while you focus on your bodily sensations.

While practicing Mindfulness Meditation, remember to focus only on the process and not on the end result. If your thoughts wander to something else such as a "to-do list" just observe that and then gently steer your focus back to the present moment and your body. The negative sensations in your body as well as your negative state of your mind should neutralize or disappear. You will be at peace.

Chapter 7

Seeing a CBT-trained Sleep Specialist

If you have not made enough progress with CBT-I, by yourself or with a therapist, you should seek the help of a sleep specialist. The "National Sleep Foundation" website www.sleepfoundation.org gives information about finding a sleep specialist. Many are associated with major hospitals. You can also find an accredited sleep specialty center that employs sleep specialist professionals by consulting the website of the American Academy of Sleep Medicine "aasmnet.org".

Within these centers, individuals who specialize in insomnia treatment or are trained in behavioral sleep medicine techniques are very likely to be able to assist you. You can also find a list of providers who are certified in behavioral sleep medicine at "absm.org/BSMSpecialists.aspx".

You may need as few as three sessions or as many as ten sessions, depending on your sleep expert, the program, and your progress. When calling to set up an appointment, ask the practitioner about his or her approach and what to expect. It is also a good idea to check ahead of time whether your health insurance will cover the treatment you need. By seeing a sleep specialist, you may find that you have another sleep disorder which has gone undetected--such as sleep apnea.

If, after seeing a sleep specialist, you still suffer from chronic insomnia, you may need to be screened for some other medical or psychiatric condition that is preventing you from getting restful sleep (such as fibromyalgia, bipolar disorder, schizophrenia, or schizo-affective disorder). If you have any of these disorders, you might need medication for sleep. If this happens to be the case, there is certainly no need for you to view this need as some kind of failure or disaster. In the end, there is a viable solution for every case of insomnia.

References

1. **Schute, N.** (2014). Working With A Therapist Can Help When Sleeping Pills Don't. *shots. www.npr.org.,* Feb. 14.

2. **American Sleep Association.** (2007). About Insomnia. American Sleep Association™ ©2015. *www.sleepassociation.org*, Sept.

3. **Smith, MT., Perlis, ML.** (2006). Who is a candidate for cognitive-behavioral therapy for insomnia? *Health Psychol.*, 25 (1), 15-9.

4. **Winehouse, B.** (2015). Sounding the Alarm on Sleep. *Reader's Digest*, Vol.185, Iss.1108, 130-137.

5. **Colton, HR., Altevogt, BM.** (Eds.). (2006). *Sleep Disorders and Sleep Deprivation: An Unmet Public Health Problem.* Institute of Medicine (US) Committee on Sleep Medicine and Research; Washington (DC): National Academies Press, Chapter 3.

6. **Adams, A.** (2010). Insomnia: The Hidden Epidemic. *The National Recovery Plan Ezine*, Iss.6.

7. **Hemp, P.** (2004). Presenteeism: At Work-But out of It. *Harvard Business Review Magazine*, Oct.1.

8. **Hetter, K.** (2018). This is the world's happiest country in 2018. CNN travel® *cnn.com/travel* ©2020 Cable News Network. A Warner Media Company. All rights Reserved. CNN Sans™ & ©2016 Cable News Network.

9. **Lazarus, CN.** (2014). Four Habits of Happy People. *Psychology Today*, Jan.17.

10. **Tuck.** How Much Sleep Does a Person Need? *www.tuck.com* July 18, 2019 Tuck®.

11. **Kelso, CM., Gentili, A., Fernandez, A.; Ahmed I, Talavera, F. (Eds.).** (2014). Primary Insomnia. *Medscape* www.emedicine.medscape.com., WebMD® LLC 1994-2015, Aug.25.

12. **Reddy, MS., Chakrabarty, A.** (2011). "Comorbid" Insomnia. *Indian J Psychol Med.*, 33(1), 1-4.

13. **Morin, CM, Culbert JP, Schwartz, SM.** (1994). Nonpharmacological interventions for insomnia: a meta-analysis of treatment efficiency. *Am J Psychiatry,* Aug;151(8): 1172-80.

14. **Morin, CM., Beaulieu-Bonneau S., Ivers, H., Vallieres, A., Guay, B., Savard, J., & Merette, C.** (2014). Speed and trajectory changes of insomnia symptoms during acute treatment with cognitive -behavioral therapy, singly and combined with medication. *Sleep Medicine,* 15(6), 701-707. doi: 10.1016/*j.sleep.* 2014.02.004.02.004. Epub. (2014), Mar.31.

15. **Cuijpers, P., Morin, CM., Lancee, J., van Straten, A., van der Zweerde, T., Kleiboer, A.** (2018). Cognitive and behavioral therapies in the treatment of insomnia: A meta-analysis. *Sleep Med Rev,* Apr;38: 3-16. Doi: 10.1016/j.smrv.2017.02.001. Epub 2017 Feb.9.

16. **Jansson-Frojmark, Norell-Clarke, A.** (2016). Cognitive Behavioral Therapy for Insomnia in Psychiatric Disorders. *Curr Sleep Med Rep.*, 2(4): 233-240. doi: 10.1007/s40675-016-0055-y. Published online 2016 Oct.20.

17. **Cunningham, JEA., Shapiro, CM.** (2018). Cognitive-Behavioural Therapy for Insomnia (CBT-I) to treat depression: A systematic review. *J Psychsom Res.* Mar; 106: 1-12. doi: 10.1016/j.psychores.2017.12.012. Epub 2017 Dec.24.

18. **Ho, FY., Chung, KF., Young., WF, Ng, TH., Kwan, KS., Yung, KP., & Cheng, SK.** (2015). Self-help Cognitive-behavioral therapy for insomnia: a meta-analysis of randomized controlled trials. *Sleep Med Rev.*, 19: 17-28. doi: 0.1016/*j.smrv*.2014.03.010. Epub. (2014), Jul.9.

19. **Harris, SF.** (2010). Overcoming Insomnia Without Drugs. *The New York Times (nytimes.com).*, Jul.8.

20. **Lader, MH.** (1999). Limitations on the use of benzodiazepines in anxiety and insomnia: are they justified? E*ur Neuropsychopharmacol.*, Suppl 6: 5399-405.

21. **Benca, RM.** (2005). Diagnosis and treatment of chronic insomnia: a review. *Psychiatr Serv.*, 56(3), 332-43.

22. **Kravitz, RL.** (2000). Direct-to-consumer advertising of prescription drugs. *West J Med.*, 173(4), 221-222.

23. **Elliott, C.** (2006). The Drug Pushers. *The Atlantic.* April Issue.

24. **Lader, MH.** (2011). Benzodiazepines revisited—will we ever learn. *Addiction.*, 106(12), 2086-109. doi: 10.1111/j. 13600443.2011.03563.X. Epub 2011, Oct.17.

25. **Uzun, S., Kozumplik, O., Jakovljević, M., & Sedić, B.** (2010). Side effects of treatment with benzodiazepines. *Psychiatr. Danub.*, 22(1), 90-3.

26. **Lalive, AL., Rudolph, U., Löscher, C., & Tan, KR.** (2011). Is there a way to curb benzodiazepine addiction? *Swiss Med Wkly.* Oct.19, 141: w13277. doi: 10.4414/smw.2011.13277.

27. **Lader, M.** (2011). Benzodiazepines revisited—will we ever learn. *Addiction.*, 106(12), 2086-109. doi: 10.1111/j. 13600443.2011.03563.X. Epub 2011, Oct.17.

28. **Grohol, JM.** (2014). Top 25 Psychiatric Medication Prescriptions for 2013. PsychCentral®, (*www.psychcentral.com)*, Copyright © Psych Central, May 18.

29. **Stewart, SA.** (2005). The effects of benzodiazepines on cognition. *J Clin Psychiatry.*, 66 Suppl 2:9-13.

30. **Ballokova, A., Peel, NM., Fiavola, D., Scott, IA., Gray, LC., Hubbard, RE.** (2014). Use of benzodiazepines and association with falls in older people admitted to hospital: a prospective cohort study. *Drugs Aging.,* Apr; 31 (4): 299-310. doi: 1D.1DD7/s40266-014-0159-3.

31. **Hu, X.** (2011). Benzodiazepine withdrawal seizures and management. *J Okla State Med As*

32. **Ramakrishnan, K., Scheid, DC.** (2007). Treatment options for insomnia. *Am Fam Physician*, Aug.15; 76(4): 517-26.

33. **Heydari, M., Isfeedvajani, MS.** (2013). Zolpidem dependence, abuse, and withdrawal: A case report. *J Res Med Sci.,* 18(11), 1006-7.

34. **Greenblatt, DJ., Roth, T.** (2012). Zolpidem for insomnia. Expert Opin Pharmacotherapy, Apr; 13(6): 879-93. doi: 10.1517/14656566.2012.667074. Epub 2012. March 19. Review.

35. **Mitchell, MD., Gehrman, P., Perlis, M., & Umscheid, CA.** (2012). Comparative effect of cognitive behavioral therapy for insomnia: a systematic review. *BMG Fam Prac.,* 13:40. doi: 10.1186.1471-2296-13-40.

36. **Anderson, KN.** (2018). Insomnia and cognitive behavioral therapy-how to access your patient and why it should be a standard part of care. *J Thorac Dis.,* Jan;10(Suppl 1): S94-S102. doi: 10.21037/jtd.2018.01.35.

37. **Sánchez-Ortuño, MM., Edinger, JD.** (2012). Cognitive behavioral therapy for the management of insomnia comorbid with mental disorders. *Curr Psychiatry Rep.,* 14(5), 519-28. doi: 10.1007/s11920-012-0312-9.

38. **Kaplan KA., Harvey, AG.** (2013). Behavioral treatment of insomnia in bipolar disorder. *Am J Psychiatry,*170(7): 716-20. doi:

10.1176/appi.ajp.2013, 12050708.

39. **Neckelmann, D., Mykletun, A., & Dahl, A.** (2007). Chronic Insomnia as a Risk Factor for Developing Anxiety and Depression. *Sleep*, 30(7), 873-880.

40. **Watson, D., Clark, LA., Weber, K., Assenheimer, JS., Strauss, ME., & McCormick, RA.** (1995a.). Testing a tripartite model: I. Evaluating the convergent and discriminant validity of anxiety and depression symptom scales. *J. Abnor. Psychol.*, 104, 3-14.

41. **Watson, D., Clark, LA., Weber, K., Assenheimer, JS., Strauss, ME., & McCormick, RA.** (1995b.). Testing a tripartite model: II. Exploring the symptom structure of anxiety and depression in student, adult, and patient samples. *J. Abnor. Psychol.*, 104, 15-25.

42. **Clark, LA., Watson, D.** (1991b.). Tripartite model of anxiety and depression: Psychometric evidence and taxonomic implications. *J. Abnor. Psychol.*, 100, 316 -36.

43. **Alloy, LB., Kelly, Ka., Mineka, S., & Clements, CM.** (1990). *Cormorbidity in anxiety and depressive disorders: A helplessness/hopelessness perspective.* **Maser, JD., Cloninger, CR., (Eds.).** *Comorbidity in anxiety and mood disorders.* 499-543. Washington DC: American Psychiatric Press.

44. **Carrasco, JL., Diaz-Marsa, M., Saiz-Ruiz, J.** (2000). Sertraline in the treatment of mixed anxiety and depression disorder. *J Affect Disord.,* Jul; 59(1): 67-9.

45. **Stress Management Society®.** Exercise, *www.stress.org.uk/exercise.aspx.*

46. **2015 National Sleep Foundation©.** (2013). National Sleep Foundation Poll Finds Exercise Key to Good Sleep, *www.sleepfoundation.org,* Washington, D.C., March 4.

47. **Wicks, L.** (2019). Walking this much every day could reduce your dementia risk. *www.cookinglight.com.,* Copyright © Meredith Corporation. 2019, July 03.

48. **Larun, L., Brurberg, KG., Odgaard-Jensen, J., & Price, JR.** (2015). Exercise therapy for chronic fatigue syndrome. *Cochrane Database Syst Rev.,*10;2:D003200. doi: 10.1002/14651858. CD003200. Pub3.

49. **Lucy.** June 15, 2015. *Tolstoy Therapy Newsletter (www.tolstoytherapy.com).*

50. **Taylor, SE., Brown, JD.** (1988). Illusion and well-being: a social psychological perspective on mental health. *Psychol Bull.* Mar;1 03(2): 193-210.

51. **Goleman, D.** (1987). Mental Health; Trying to Face Reality? It May Be the Last Thing That the Doctor Orders. *The New York Times www.nytimes.com.,* Nov.26.

52. **Ozbay, F., Johnson, DC., Dimorlas, E., Morgan III, CA., Charney, D., Southwick, S.** (2007). *Psychiatry Edgmont.* May;4(5): 35-40.

53. **Bochard, TJ.** (2010). Spirituality and Prayer Relieve Stress. PsychCentral® *www.psychcentral.com.* Copyright © 1995-2015 Psych Central, Mar. 21.

54. **Holmes, B., Kleiner, K., Douglas, K., Bond, M.** (2004). 10 Keys to True Happiness. *Reader's Digest.,* (from *New Scientist*). March. pp.100.

55. **Briggs, J.** (2010) Exploring the Power of Meditation. National Center for Complementary and Integrative Health. Director's Page, June 25.

56. **Bertone, HJ.** (2017). Which Type of Meditation Is Right for Me? *Healthline Media® www.healthline.com.* Copyright © 2005-2019 Healthline Media, Jun.9.

57. **Rapaport, L.** (2019). Many Sleepless Americans Trying Meditation and Yoga. *Reuters Health® www.reuters.com.* Copyright ©Reuters Health,Feb.25.

58. **Voiβ, P., Hoxtermann, MD., Dobos, G., Cramer, H.** (2019). The use of mind-body medicine among U.S. individuals with sleep problems: analysis of the 2017 National Health Interview Survey data. *Sleep Med.* Apr; 56: 151-156. doi: 10.1016/j.sleep.2019.01.008. Epub 2019 Jan.18.

59. **Leavitt, J. M.ED.** (2018). 9 Breathing Exercises for Sleep: Techniques That Work. Healthline Media® *www.healthline.com* Nov.1.

60. **Newport, F.** (2016). Five Key Findings on religion in the U.S. Gallup® *news.gallup.com* Dec.23.

61. **Noonan, P.** (2004). Keeping the Faith. *Reader's Digest.,* March. pp.88.

62. **Peale, N.V.** (1996). The Power of Positive Thinking. Ballantine Books. Reissue edition: Aug.1 1996.

63. **Byrd, RC.** (1988). Positive therapeutic effects of intercessory prayer in a coronary care unit population. *South Med J.,* 81(7), 826-9.

64. **Nelson. T.** (2014). Bestselling Jesus Calling® brand celebrates 10 years and 10 million sold. Cision® PR Newswire. *www.prnewswire.com* Mar. 17.

65. **Fiallo, J.** (2019). U.S. falls in world happiness report, Finland named happiest country. *tampabay.com/data* Tampa Bay Times ©2020 All Rights Reserved. Mar. 20.

66. **Gamaldo, C.** (2020). Exercising for Better Sleep. *hopkinsmedicine.org* John Hopkins Medicine® Copyright © 2020 The John Hopkins University, The John Hopkins Hospital, and John Hopkins Health System. All Rights Reserved.

67. **Tolle, E.** (2001). Practicing The Power of Now. New World Library.

68. **Warren, R.** (2002). The Purpose Driven Life. Zandervan.

Made in the USA
Monee, IL
04 November 2022

17098512R10055